CARROTS? LET ME EXPLAIN

"Everything you need to know - and then some..."

Pearl Robinson

Copyright©2015

PEARL ROBINSON

DISCLAIMER

This book is not intended as a substitute for the medical advice of physicians. The reader should regularly consult a physician in matters relating to his/her health and particularly with respect to any symptoms that may require diagnosis or medical attention.

Table of Contents

INTRODUCTION:
WHY SHOULD YOU READ THIS eBOOK?

This eBook brings to you all you wanted to know about carrots and much more. You might think you know quite everything about the carrot as this is a popular vegetable seen and eaten in almost every other meal—at breakfast, lunch, dinner and in-between snacks.

But this seemingly regular vegetable has many secrets that will delight you. Did you know that carrots come in the colour of the rainbow? Did you know that carrots were once upon a time used exclusively as medicine? Did you know that carrots are one of the most effective natural insecticides? Did you know that carrots can be as addictive as coffee and even give you withdrawal symptoms?

Carrots are even today used as medicine as its amazing constituents provide immense health benefits. You will learn about the many traditional cures that you can use in your day-to-day life to promote your well-being. While every remedy given in this eBook is tried and tested, it is very important that you do not apply any of these remedies without consulting your doctor first.

Surprised a little? You will learn many things about your favourite vegetable in this eBook. Right from its origin to the present day, there is a lot of information packed within, which will reassure you, delight you, enlighten you and guide you.

Stay healthy and have fun reading this eBook. Thank you for downloading it.

CHAPTER 1:
CARROT - WHAT IS THIS?

A Brief History

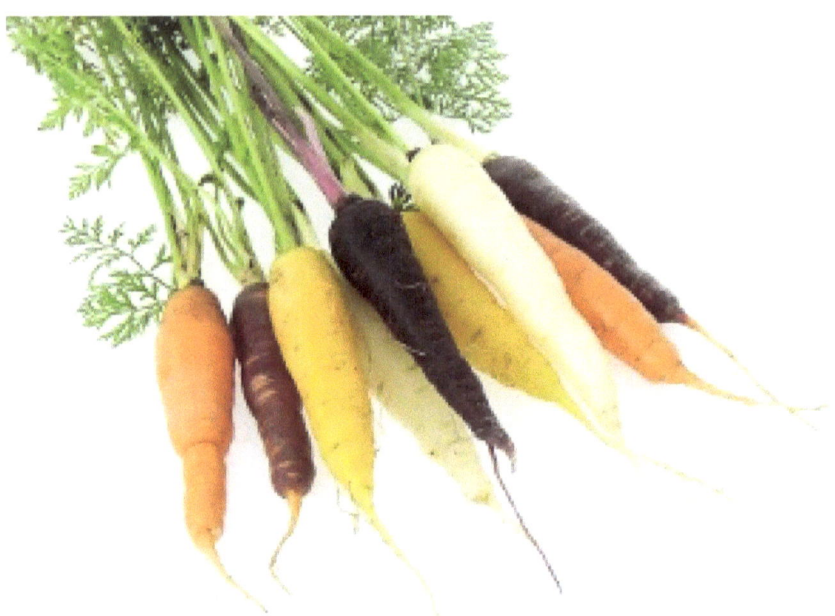

The carrot—*Daucus carota*—is a taproot native to Europe and south-western Asia. Almost half of the world's produce, which is about 35.65 million tons, comes from China. The name *"carrot"* originates from the Greek word, *"karoton"*, which means "horn-like" referring to the tapering-to-a-point shape of the vegetable.

Records show that the wild carrot originates from Persia (today's Afghanistan, Pakistan and Iran regions), where it was found about 5,000 years ago. It's still growing wild in abundance in these areas. The earliest mention dates it around 1st century—and at that time the root was yellow and purple. A quick timeline will indicate how it spread in the world until the 18th century:

➢ **Before 900 – 1000 AD** – it is grown wild in Afghanistan, Iran and North Arabia. The carrot variety is mainly purple and yellow.

➢ **1000 – 1100 AD** – It is found in North Africa, Syria and Spain; red colour carrot is added to the previous two colours.

➢ **1100 – 1300 AD** – The carrot cultivation has spread to China, Italy, The Netherlands, Germany, and France. The white colour carrot is added to the earlier repertoire.

➢ **1300 – 1500 AD** – Cultivation steadily spreads to Northern Europe where the carrot is red, white, and yellow in colour.

➢ **1500 – 1700 AD** – The carrot finds its way to Japan and North America. The colours of the carrots cultivated are red, orange, yellow and purple.

The carrot was well known and popular among Greeks and Romans. In those days, it was believed that it had properties which made women more yielding sexually. By the 13th century, the carrot became common as a food crop in Asia, particularly in China, Japan, and India.

Europe did not have this vegetable until the Middle Ages where it was used more medicinally than as a culinary delight. It first arrived in England in the Elizabethan Era, when it was used as food, medicine and decoration for hats, hair and dresses of the ladies at Court. During this time, carrots were often interchanged in name and use with their cousin, parsnips.

The modern carrot—as we know it today—is the result of extensive selective cultivation aimed at minimizing, if not totally eliminating, its innate bitter taste and wooden core.

Vegetable or Fruit

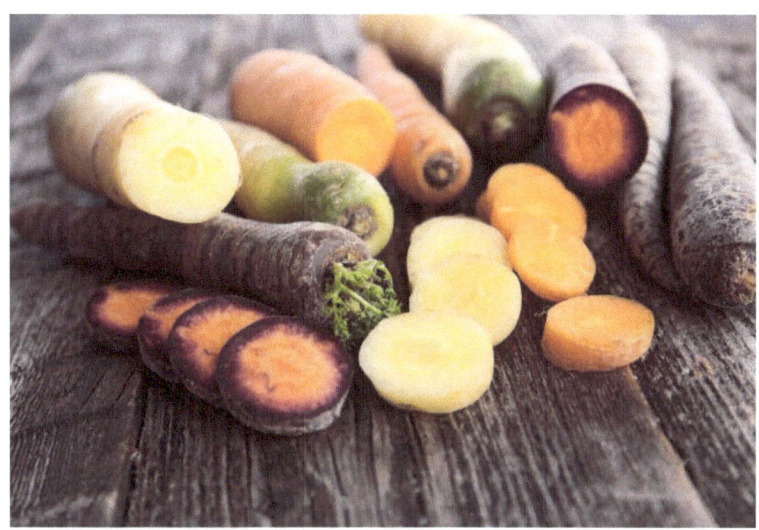

We all know that the tomato is a fruit, though we use it as a vegetable. What about the carrot? Is it a fruit or vegetable? The 2001 European Union Jam Directive lists the carrot as a fruit. It is believed that this was done to favor the Portuguese, who are fixated on carrot marmalade (see recipe at the end of the book).

"Marmalade" by the way is British terminology. It is used for any jam that contains citrus fruit with the peel—hence, the customary British orange marmalade, which is sweet with a tinge of bitter.

By scientific definition, the carrot is a vegetable, i.e. part of a plant grown for food, which is not formed out of a flower, nor contains seeds. This is how the tomato is defined scientifically as a fruit, i.e. it develops from a flower and contains seeds.

CHAPTER 2: VARIETIES OF CARROTS

The Wild Carrot of Today

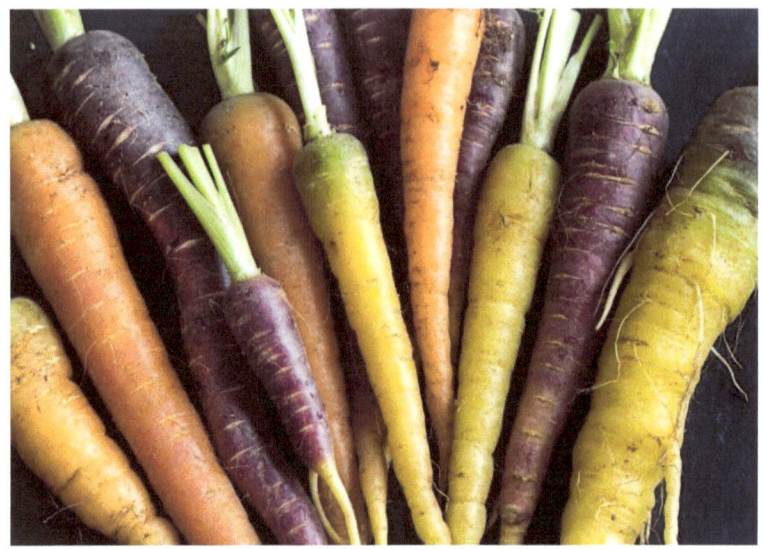

The Peruvian Carrot

This is a related-to-carrot variety popularly known as the *"Peruvian carrot"* or *"Arracacia xanthorriza"*, which originated in the Andes. A major commercial crop in Brazil, South America this looks like a cross between celery and carrot. The root is short and thick covered with off-white shiny skin and the inside can be purple, yellow or white. The leaves, which look very much like parsley in shape can be purple or dark green.

The Sea Carrot

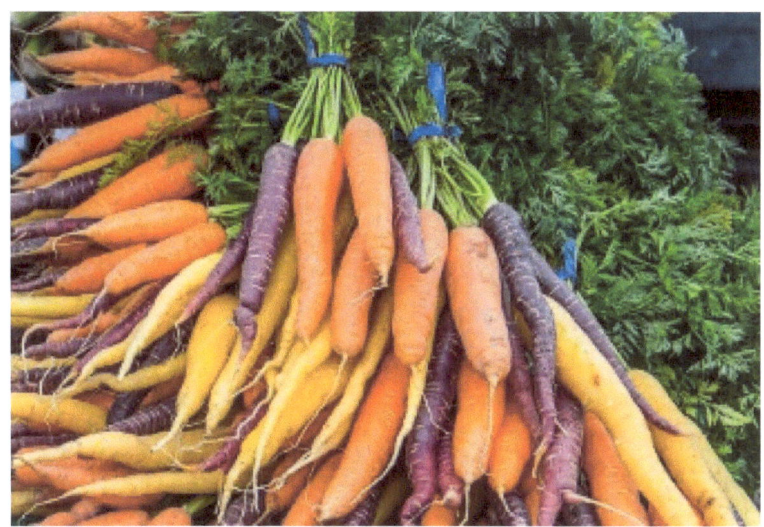

Also known as *Dacus carota gummifera*, this is a carrot species that grows wild in the British Isles. It is found mostly around the coast, almost under the sea—from where it derives its name. The plant has thick succulent stems, dark green leaves, and lilac coloured flower umbels.

Types of Carrots: By Colour

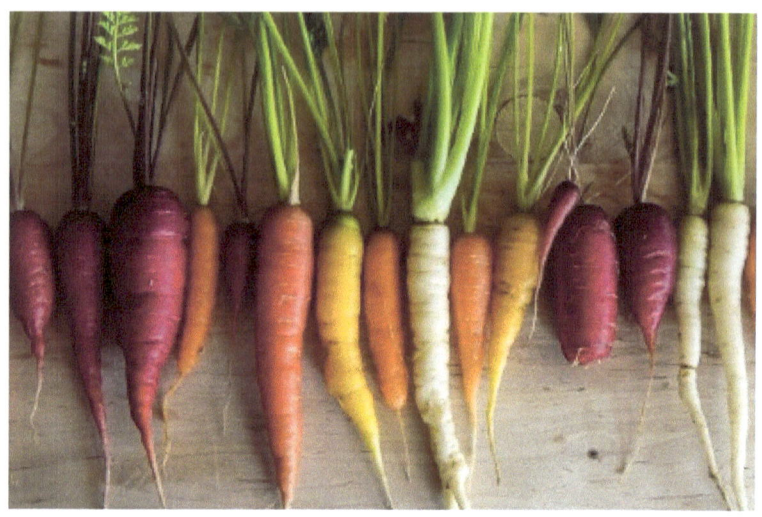

It is a little known fact that carrots come in many colours. Most people know the carrot as the yellow-orange vegetable. From its Afghanistan ancestry, the carrot spread to the East and West and developed different characteristics. In the east, it spread to Japan and India through north Asia; this cultivar was mostly red. In the west, the cultivar was mostly yellow, and then changed to orange.

The original colour of the ancestor of this vegetable was purple/black. Through its journey over the world, it mutated and changed into a number of colours, i.e. black, orange, purple, red white and yellow—each genotype slightly different in contents and properties.

Black Carrots

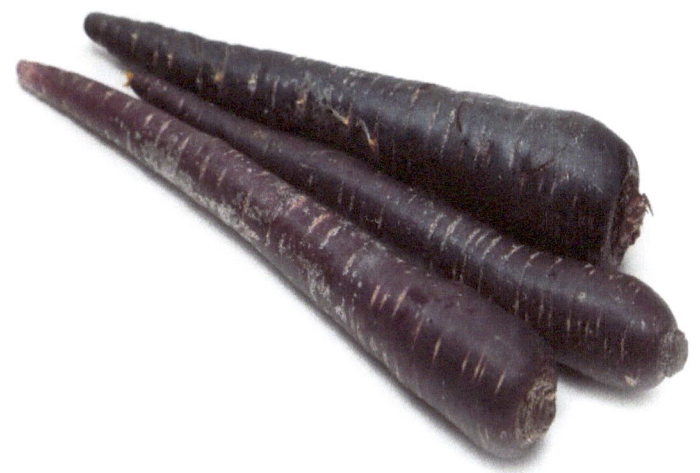

Black carrots genetics clearly show descendancy from the Eastern genotype that can be traced to Turkey and Syria. This carrot is an exceptionally rich source of anthocyanins, flavonols, B-carotene, phenols and minerals such as zinc, iron, and calcium. The advantage of the black carrot over its orange counterpart is that its antioxidant properties are 28 times higher.

The black carrot is sweet and rich in taste. It can be eaten raw or cooked, and it's best used in salads as pickle and juiced.

The juice of the black carrot is used as a blood cleanser and for treating stomach disorders, constipation, skin pigmentation, and acne. It is also good for eyesight and blood circulation. This will tone and moisturize the skin.

Orange Carrots

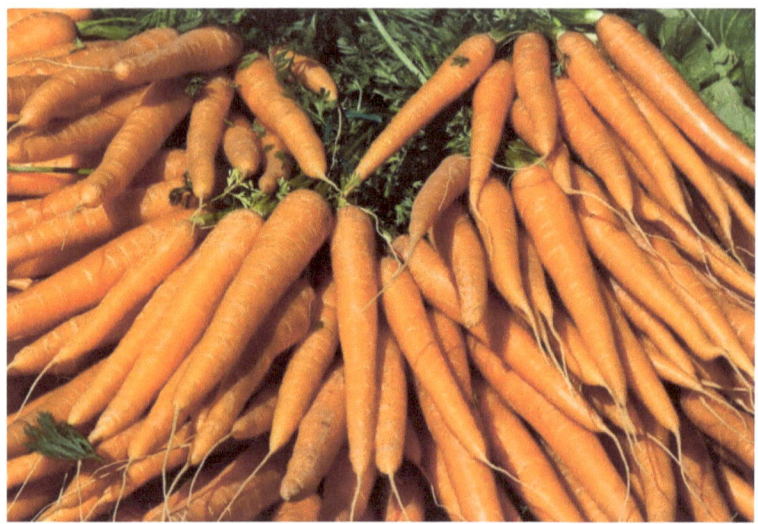

This is the carrot that we know today; the most popular in the modern world. It originates from the Middle East and Europe. Its colour is derived from the rich content of beta-carotene and alpha-carotene, which is highly beneficial for the health of eyes. It is also the primary factor that improves night sight. The orange pigment helps produce rhodopsin, a key component that increases light sensitiveness in the retina.

Some examples of orange carrot varieties are Top Cut, Sirkana, Navajo, Danvers, and Scarlet Nantes.

Purple Carrots

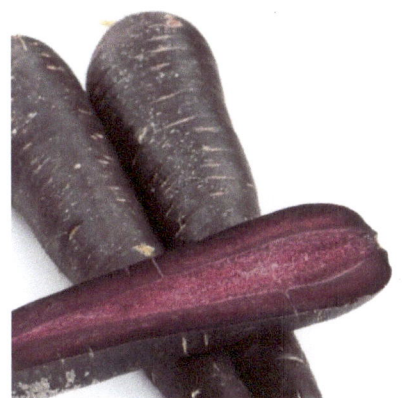 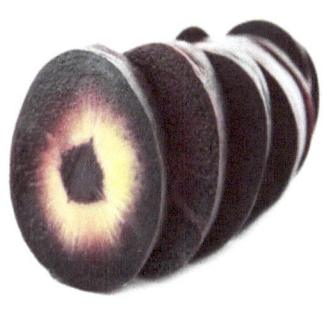

The purple carrot is the first genotype of the vegetable; the ancestor of today's modern carrot. You will find these carrots growing mostly in Asia and Europe. The colour is owed to its pH sensitive molecular structure, which changes to basic from acidic. The inside part of the purple carrot is white, orange or purple. It has a peppery flavour, but they are sweet and smooth in taste.

Among the popular varieties include Purple Haze, Cosmic Purple, Purple Dragon, Maroon, and Indigo.

The purple pigment is derived from a class of most powerful antioxidants called anthocyanins; the same that gives colour to blueberries and raspberries. The purple carrot consists of 28 times more anthocyanins than the regular (orange) carrot.

Red Carrots

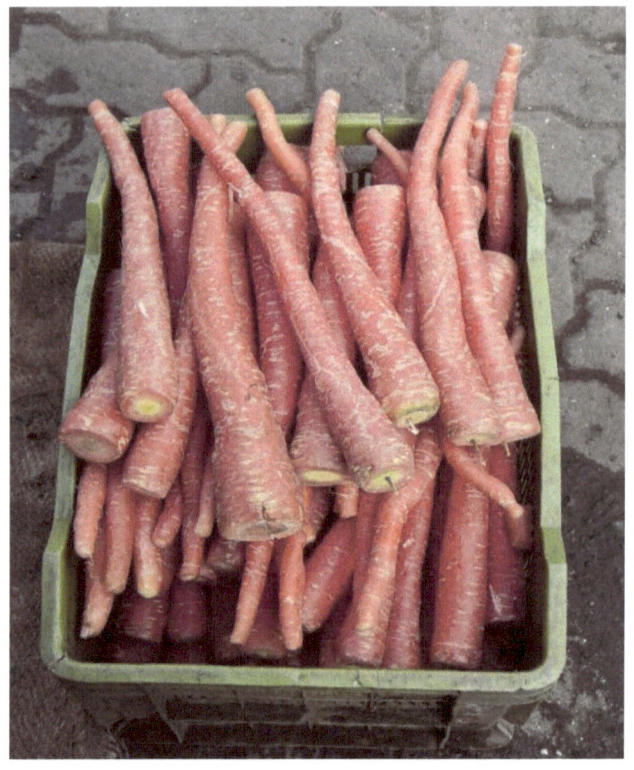

The red carrots originate from China and India and are best known for their properties that prevent cancer of the prostate. Their colour comes from a class of pigments called lycopene, which is a heart-friendly carotene. This is the same pigment that colours the tomato and watermelon. The taste is sweet and rich with an earthy flavour.

An antioxidant most abundant in the red carrot is lutein, which helps prevent macular degeneration and age-related blindness. Some popular varieties of red colour carrots are Red Samurai and Red Chateney.

White or Golden Carrots

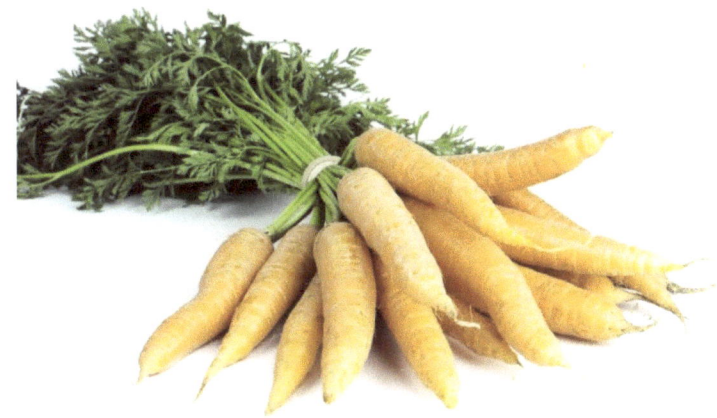

White carrots are white because of lack of pigmentation (carotene) and the presence of a recessive gene for Vitamin E (tocopherol). This is also the reason why they are believed to be less "healthy" than the orange carrot though they are still a good source of fibre and heart-friendly compounds. The taste of the white carrot is sweeter and richer than any other colour carrot.

Before the 16th century, the white carrot was mostly used as cattle fodder. Today this carrot is preferred by people who are allergic to carotene, the pigment which gives the carrot its common orange colour. Unfortunately, owing to its colour, the white carrot's history is intertwined and interchanged with that of parsnip.

Some popular varieties are White Satin and Crème de Lite.

Yellow Carrots

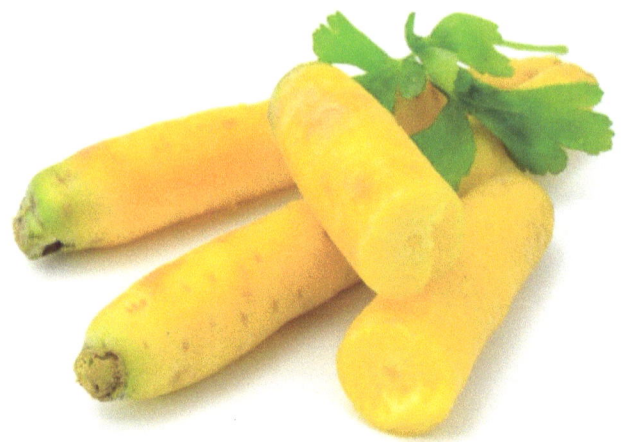

Yellow carrots owe their colour to a pigment similar to beta-carotene called xanthophylls, which is especially beneficial for healthy eyes. This is especially good for the health of the eyes and eyesight. The origins of these carrots can be traced to the Middle East. Research studies show that the yellow and red varieties are most effective foods against cardio-vascular diseases.

This genotype is very popular all over the world owing to its high resistance to pests, salinity, diseases, drought and heat. Some examples of varieties of yellow carrots are Yellowstone, Solar Yellow, and Sunlite.

Types of Carrots: By Varieties

The carrots types are divided into 4 major categories by their shape, i.e. the Danvers, Imperators, Nantes and Chantenay carrots.

Nantes

The Nantes carrots are the best choice for home gardening. They thrive in rocky soil, and they don't usually form pithy cores if left in the field, unlike Chantenay carrots.

➢ **Bolero** – this is a hybrid cultivar that takes about 70 days to harvest. It grows up to 8 inches in length, slightly tapered, uniformly thick and with a blunt tip. It is especially high yielding and resistant to foliage disease.

➢ **Cosmic Purple** - this cultivar takes about 73 days to harvest. It grows up to 7 inches in length, is purple-violet on the outside and bright orange inside. Unlike the majority of purple carrots, this variety retains their colour on cooking.

➢ **Ingot** - this is a hybrid cultivar that takes about 70 days. It is deep orange in colour, grows up to 8 inches long, has an indistinct core, is extremely sweet and has a strong top.

- ➤ **Nantes Coreless** – this cultivar takes about 68 days to harvest. It is orange-red in colour, has a medium top and small core.

- ➤ **Nelson** - this cultivar takes about 58 days to harvest. It is the happiest in heavy soil. It grows up to 7 inches and a total thickness of about 1 inch. It is dark orange in colour and very sweet in taste.

- ➤ **Purple Dragon** - this cultivar takes about 70 days to harvest. This is dark purple in colour on the outside and has a deep orange core; when cooked it loses its colour. A goldmine of phytochemicals for the body, this carrot grows up to 8 inches, is sweet and very tasty.

- ➤ **Scarlet Nantes** - this cultivar takes about 70 days to harvest. It is bright orange and grows up to 6 inches, it's sweet, tender, and flavourful.

- ➤ **Sweetness** - this is a hybrid cultivar that takes about 63 days. It's about 6 inches long, 1 inch thick, cylindrical and has a crunchy texture and is sweet in taste.

- ➤ **Touchon** - this cultivar takes about 63 days to harvest. It's sweet and very tasty at any size, almost coreless, bright orange both outside and inside and grows up to 7 inches.

➤ **White Satin** – this cultivar takes about 70 days to harvest. This is a white variety, with a sweet, crunchy taste. It grows up to 8 inches in length.

➤ **Yaya** - this cultivar takes about 60 days to harvest and is especially suitable for a fall sowing. A little less sweet in taste, but tender in texture.

Imperator

The Imperator variety of carrots is slim and well tapered to a thin point. It is happiest in sandy, loam soil.

➤ **Avenger** - this hybrid cultivar takes about 70 days to harvest. It grows up to 9 inches long, is slightly blunt and tapered.

   ➤

➤ **Cosmic Red** - this cultivar takes about 65-75 days to harvest. It has a bright red colour and is best consumed cooked.

➤ **Gold Pak** - this cultivar takes about 76 days to harvest. It is a coreless variety that grows up to 8 inches long and 1 ½ inches thick. It has a tender texture and sweet taste.

- ➢ **Imperator 58** - this cultivar takes about 68 days to harvest. It is thin with a long tapered root.

- ➢ **Legend** - this hybrid cultivar takes about 68 days to harvest. It grows up to 11 inches long and 1 ½ inches thick.

- ➢ **Orlando Gold** - this hybrid cultivar takes about 78 days to harvest. It has an excellent flavour and bright colour owed to about 30% more carotene. It has a beautifully tapered shape.

- ➢ **Sugarsnax 54** - this cultivar takes about 68 days to harvest. It has a beautiful red-orange colour owing to its rich beta-carotene content. It grows up to 9 inches long and is resistant to Cercospora blights and Altenaria.

- ➢ **Tendersweet** - this cultivar takes about 75 days to harvest. It's rich orange in colour, coreless and sweet.

Chantenay

This variety is a favorite for gardeners because it is a tough lot that grows well in difficult terrains. Before the Nantes variety was developed and popularized, this variety was the sole option for gardeners who had clay and rocky soil. They need to be harvested when they are about 6-7 inches as the older carrots tend to develop a woody core.

➤ **Hercules** - this cultivar takes about 65 days to harvest. This is especially good for soils that are rocky/clay where other carrot varieties are unable to thrive.

➤ **Red-Cored Chantenay** - this cultivar takes about 70 days to harvest. It has a sweet and rich flavour, it's short and thick, and it tapers to a blunt tip. It retains its sweetness in storage.

➤ **Royal Chantenay** - this cultivar takes about 70 days to harvest. This is bright orange with a broad top and tapered tips.

Danvers

➤ **Danvers Half-Long** - this cultivar takes about 75 days to harvest. It grows up to 8 inches in length, it's tender and sweet and has a blunt end.

➤ **Danvers 126** - this cultivar takes about 75 days to harvest. It gives a heavier yield than the Danvers and can withstand heat better.

In addition to these four categories, there are three more special varieties, i.e. Novelty, Baby and Small and Round carrots.

Novelty Carrots

➢ **Belgium White** – it takes about 75 days to harvest. They are golden to white, tapered, sweet with a mild flavour.

Baby Carrots

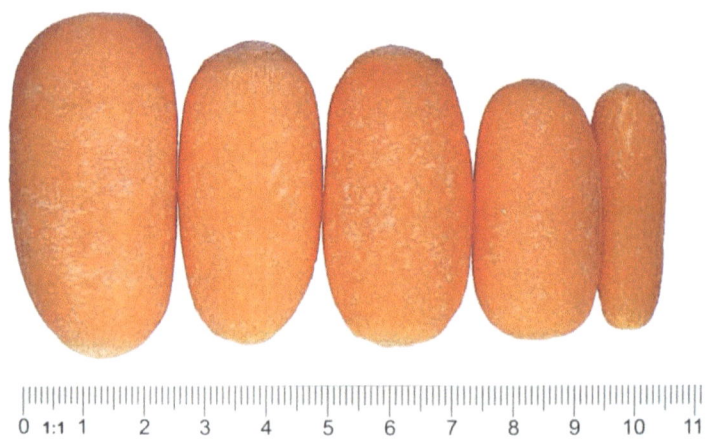

Baby carrots are a recent addition to the list of "*carrot types*". A California farmer is credited with the "discovery" of the baby carrot concept. These carrots are not a particular/special variety, but the young version of carrots, which easily explains the tiny size and tender texture. The use of baby carrots as healthy snacks was an idea promoted by California carrot farmers in 2010.

Small size carrots, however, do exist and these varieties grow best in regions with shallow and rocky soil because they do not need depth to grow.

➤ **Thumbelina** – it takes about 60 days to harvest. They require rocky, shallow soil and are excellent for container planting.

➤ **Orbit** – it takes about 58 days to harvest. It is flattish, the size of 50 cents and sweet.

➤ **Babette** - this cultivar takes about 55 days to harvest. It grows up to 4 inches. It is served in high-end restaurants with the tops attached. It's crunchy, rich in taste and sweet.

➤ **Romeo** - this cultivar takes about 65 days to harvest. It grows up to 2 inches long, spherical, like a radish, bright orange and sweet.

CHAPTER 3: USE OF CARROTS

Cooked Vs Raw Carrot

This could seem an odd question to someone who is used to the basic concept that cooking kills the majority of nutrients in vegetables. With carrots, however, it is exactly the opposite. Since the nutrition wealth is trapped within protein sacks in the carrot, processing it through heating, juicing, grinding and even chewing increases the nutrient value of this vegetable.

Steaming the carrots, juicing or pureeing will increase the availability of the carotenoids—the beneficial compounds of the carrot—by a whopping 600%. Cooking carrots in healthy fat/oil increases the absorption of carotenoids into the blood by a mind-boggling 1000%. This is because carotenoids are fat-soluble compounds.

While eating carrots raw is still good for the body, in the case of this vegetable, it looks like cooking it increases its value to the body exponentially.

Carrot is excellent in smoothies and as juice. To improve the assimilation of the beneficial nutrients in the body, add about ½ a teaspoon of virgin olive oil per glass of juice/smoothie.

Storing Carrots At Home

Fresh Carrots

Fresh carrots can be stored in the refrigerator for weeks if stored right and purchased fresh. Trim the leaves as soon as you can as they pull away the moisture from the carrot. Store the carrots in dry plastic ziplock bags in the crisper part of your fridge. You may store them whole, diced, sliced or julienned.

Canned Carrots

To can carrots is very simple, and you will be assured of a good source of your favorite vegetable whenever you need it. Follow these 5 simple steps:

➢ Select small size carrots; maximum about 1 ½ inch thick. Peel, wash and dice or slice.

➢ Heat a saucepan and add water and the carrots to it. The water level should be just above the carrots.

➢ Boil the water on high heat. Reduce the heat and simmer for about 5 minutes.

➢ Transfer the carrots into hot jars filling it up to 1 inch from the top. Fill with boiling water and add ½ spoon of salt/pint.

> ➤ Remove all air bubbles and wipe dry the rims of the jar. Place the 2-piece lids and process.

> ➤ Process at 11 pounds pressure in a Dial Gauge Pressure Canner or at 10 pounds pressure in a Weighted Gauge Pressure for 25 minutes for a pint or 30 minutes for a quart.

Frozen Carrots

Choose young, small size, tender carrots; maximum about 1 ½ inch thick and blanch them. This ensures that the enzyme activity is slowed down or completely stopped, which helps retain the colour, texture and flavour of the carrot. Follow the steps given below:

> ➤ Cut the carrots into 1/4 inch cubes, thin slices/strips. The small carrots you could use whole.

> ➤ Blanch the diced carrots for about 2 minutes, whole carrots for 6 minutes and those cut into strips for about 2 minutes.

> ➤ Transfer to cold water and leave for 5 minutes. Drain and place in packets leaving about ½ inch space.

> ➤ Seal and deep freeze.

Cooking With Carrots

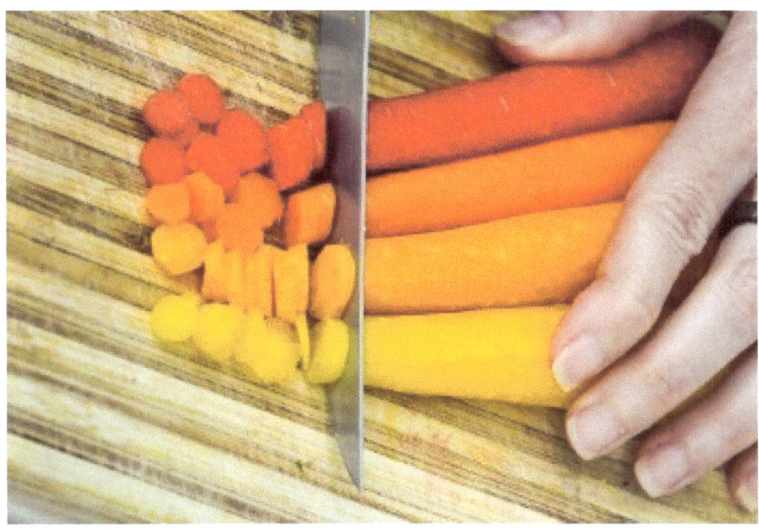

There are many ways to use carrots while cooking. In fact, cooked carrots are actually healthier than raw carrots. Hence, it makes sense to learn ways you can cook this remarkable vegetable. The good thing about carrots is that they are versatile and have a virtually indestructible structure, which gives you total freedom to experiment your culinary talents.

One important tip you should keep in mind when you use and/or store carrots is that you need to keep them away from pears, apples and potatoes. The proximity to these foods will make the carrots bitter.

The Basics of Cooking Carrots

Carrots need to be cooked according to their age. It is very important that you use carrots of trusted origins. Carrots are best eaten with their skin as it is the skin that holds the best of the nutrients. Hence, as much as possible you should use carrots without peeling them.

➤ Young carrots are the best, usually available early summer. This type of carrot requires very little preparation. Do not peel them; just rinse them thoroughly in water and cook whole. You may blanch them with ½ teaspoon of olive oil or butter. These are best for salads and grilling.

➤ Older carrots, which are also known as main crop carrots are best for stews, soups and casseroles. You may like to dice, slice and julienne these carrots, which can be boiled, steamed, grilled and sautéed for best taste and flavour.

➤ Old carrots tend to develop a woody core hence, if you are using this type for cooking, use the outer parts and discard the core. These are best in soups and stews. You can also grate these carrots for cooking desserts.

10 Ways to Cook Carrots

1. Blanching Carrots
- Clean the carrots
- Place a pot of water on high heat and bring to boil.
- Boil the carrots for about 5-6 minutes. If they are older boil for about 10-12 minutes.

2. Steaming Carrots
- Use a steamer machine and follow the instructions.
- If you are using a saucepan or steaming basket, ensure that the water level is below the steamer that holds the carrots.
- Bring water to boil.
- Cover with the lid and continue boiling the water for about 15 minutes.

3. Boiled Carrots
- This is especially recommended for old carrots. Instead of water, you may use vegetable or chicken stock.
- Slice or dice the carrots as required.
- Add water and salt to a saucepan and bring to a boil.
- Reduce heat and add the carrots.
- Boil on low heat for about 10 minutes.

4. Microwave Carrots

- Clean the carrots (about 1lb) and place in a microwave dish.
- Microwave on high until the carrots are tender and crisp.
- For timing, thin slices will take about 9 minutes, strips 7 minutes and baby carrots about 9 minutes.

5. Braised Carrots

- The oven needs to be preheated to 275 degrees Fahrenheit (in Celsius it's 140 degrees).
- Prepare 1lb. of carrots as per your requirements, i.e. slice, dice, julienne or use baby carrots as whole.
- Place the carrots flat in a Dutch oven or casserole pot.
- Add to the carrots 1/3 cup of extra virgin olive oil, 2 tsp orange zest, 1/3 cup shallots diced and 1¼ cups of orange juice.
- Place the pot on the stove at medium heat and bring to a boil. Once it starts boiling, remove from heat and cover with a lid. If you do not have a lid, use with heavy kitchen foil for this purpose.
- Place the pot in the oven and cook for 1½ hours or until tender.

6. Glazed Carrots

- Have the carrots cleaned and sliced.
- Steam for about 8 minutes.
- Place a pan on heat and melt 25g of butter in it. Add to the melted butter ½ cup of sugar.
- Add 2 tbsp orange juice to this mix and toss the carrots in. Continue to cook for about 1 minute and remove from heat.
- Use chopped nuts and fresh parsley for garnishing.

7. Roasted Carrots

- Quarter carrots and keep them aside.
- Brush the carrots with olive oil or melted butter.
- Have the oven preheated to 400 degrees Fahrenheit (In Celsius it's 200 degrees).
- Place carrots in the oven and roast for about 30 minutes. Turn the carrots a few times to ensure that you get even caramelization.

8. Stir Fried Carrots

- Prepare the carrots as per your requirements.
- Add a few teaspoons of olive oil to a saucepan and place on heat.
- Add the carrots and stir-fry on high heat until tender and crisp.
- Garnish with chopped mint.

9. Barbecued Carrots
- Slice the carrots along their length.
- Brush with olive oil or melted butter.
- Have the carrots barbecued. Remove when caramelized.

10. Pureed Carrots
- Take about 10 oz young carrots and add to salted water. Add ½ oz oil or butter to the water.
- Place on high heat and cook until tender.
- Drain the water retaining just about 1 cup for later use.
- Blend the cooked carrots with a little drained water to get carrot puree.
- Heat the puree with a little oil to make it smooth.
- To make the puree rich and creamy, add about 4 tbsp to it just before serving.

Carrot Smoothies

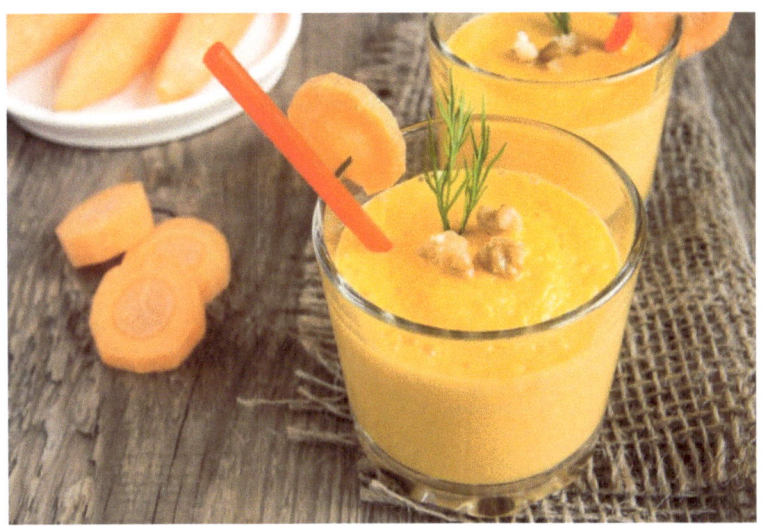

Carrots make excellent smoothies as they have a mild flavour and are a goldmine of nutrients that are better absorbed when blended. Check out some exceptional recipes for smoothies here—

http://www.incrediblesmoothies.com/recipes/carrot-smoothie-recipes-and-nutrition/

Carrot Desserts

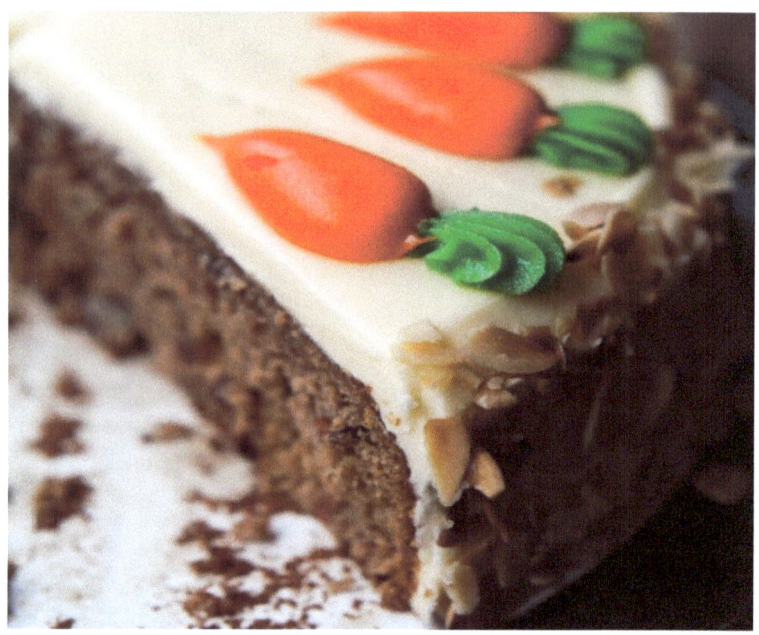

Carrots are naturally sweet and, therefore, make exceptionally good ingredients for desserts. Check out recipes for carrot halwa, carrot cake, carrot pie and carrot doughnuts.

Carrot: Alternative Medicine

A popular medicinal herb used in Traditional Chinese Medicine (TCM) system, the carrot has been identified with the following major medicinal properties:

➢ Stimulant
➢ Ophthalmic (benefits the eyes)
➢ Galactogogue (promotes lactation)
➢ Emmenagogue (stimulates menstruation blood flow)
➢ Diuretic (promotes expelling of urine)
➢ Deobstruent
➢ Contraceptive
➢ Carminative (expelling flatulence)
➢ Anthelmintic (expels and destroys worms)

For maximum benefits out of the carrot, it is recommended that you take 2-3 glasses of carrot juice per day. According to TCM, here are some quick, simple yet extremely potent remedies using carrot. The prescriptions below are reliable and trusted; nonetheless, it is highly recommended that you do not adopt any of these remedies without consulting your physician first.

Constipation Treatment

Make 2.7 ounces carrot juice, add 2-3 drops of olive oil and about 1 teaspoon of royal jelly honey. Mix well and take it once in the morning and once at night.

Hypertension Treatment

Drink about 3 ounces of carrot juice in equally divided doses once in the morning and once at night for 30 days.

Night Blindness Treatment

Sauté on slow heat about 250 grams of orange, yellow or red carrots in 2 tablespoons of olive oil until well done. Eat this along with your meal every day for 7 days.

Long-term Cough Treatment

Take 200 grams of fresh organic carrots and about 10-13 Chinese red dates and put them into a cooking pot along with 8 cups of water. Cook on slow fire for about 30 minutes. Drink this mixture once every day until the cough is gone.

Dandruff and Itchy Scalp Treatment

Take 200 grams of fresh organic carrots and stew them over low heat for about 30 minutes. Add salt to taste. Drink it once a day along with your meal.

The following are juices that are meant to help you

cure certain maladies. Please follow the instruction to the T:

➢ The juice needs to be taken for a minimum of 6 consecutive months.

➢ Use organic products exclusively. When "in-between meal time" is advised, this means about 2-3 hours before your mealtime.

➢ Do not take these remedies along with any medication—unless your doctor has advise it.

➢ Make the juice when you need to drink it as delaying it will cause certain delicate nutrients to die.

Scurvy

Blend 8 ounces each of carrots and grapefruit. Blend for 30-45 seconds at highest speed or until smooth. Have it in-between meals, once a day.

Adenoids, Acne

Take 10 ounces of carrots and 6 ounces of spinach and blend for 30-45 seconds at the highest speed or until smooth. Have it in-between meals, once a day.

Rheumatism

Take 8 ounces each of carrots and celery and blend for 30-45 seconds at the highest speed or until smooth. Have it in-between meals, once a day.

Tumors

Mix 8 ounces each of carrot and beet and blend for 30-45 seconds at the highest speed or until smooth. Have it in-between meals, once a day.

Bright's disease

Mix in blender 8 ounces of carrot, 6 ounces of celery and 2 ounces of parsley and blend for 30-45 seconds at the highest speed or until smooth. Have it in-between meals, once a day.

Dermatitis

Mix 6 ounces of carrot, 5 ounces of beet and 5 ounces of cucumber into the blender. Blend for 30-45 seconds at the highest speed or until smooth. Have it in-between meals, once a day.

Colitis

Mix 8 ounces each of carrots and apples into a blender. Blend for 30-45 seconds at the highest speed or until smooth. Have it in-between meals, once a day.

Warts

Take one carrot and grate it. Mix the grated carrot with olive oil and make a paste. Apply this paste to the wart morning and night, and cover it with a Band-Aid. The wart will disappear within 15 days.

Home Made Beauty Remedies

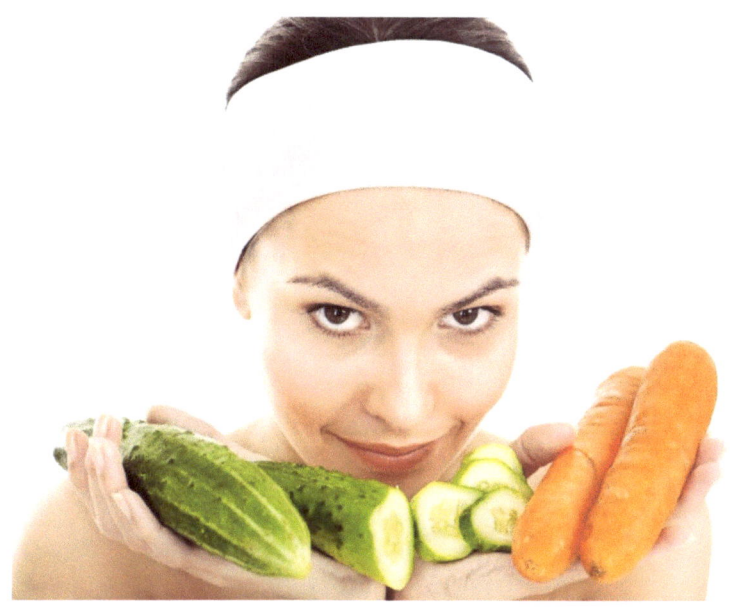

Carrots are well known for their amazing effect on skin care. Here are a few easy-to-make home remedies that will help you look gorgeous. Daily drinking carrot juice will cleanse your system and give you a glowing skin. It will insulate you from sunburn and prevent and reverse ageing signs.

Drinking carrot juice will also keep your skin moisturized, toned and free from infection. It promotes quick healing of any type of skin infections, as well.

Acne Treatment

Drinking carrot juice purifies the blood and prevents and treats acne. You may also mash raw carrot and apply on the face for 20 minutes every alternate day to clear acne and blemishes.

De-tanning Face Mask

Take equal amounts of papaya and carrot paste (both raw) and mix with 1-2 teaspoons of raw milk. Apply this mask to your face and keep for 20 minutes. Wash with warm water.

Natural Skin Moisturizer

Take a spoon each of honey and carrot juice. Apply this mix to the face and wash off after 15 minutes. Do this 3 times a week and you'll never worry about dry or dull skin.

Acne and Pimple Mask

Mix carrot juice (about 2 teaspoons) with 2 pinches of cinnamon and 1 teaspoon of honey to make thick paste. Apply this over the face for 20 minutes and wash with warm water. Besides getting rid of pimples, acne and blemishes, it will give a beautiful warm glow to your face.

Anti-ageing Mask

Take 2 tablespoons of carrot juice, add a few drops of lemon juice, a little banana pulp, and ½ egg white. Apply to the face and leave for 15-25 minutes. Wash your face first with warm water followed by a dash of cold water. This is amazing for sagging skin.

Exfoliation Mask

Take 2 tablespoons of ground-to-paste carrot and add to it 3 pinches of turmeric, 1 teaspoon gram flour and 1 teaspoon yoghurt and mix into a paste. Leave on the face for about 20 minutes and wash with cold water. This will leave your face glowing, toned and de-tanned.

CHAPTER 4: HEALTH INFORMATION

Carrot attributes with a long list of health benefits among which are:

- ➤ It fights lung infection and reduces cough in general.
- ➤ Enhances the functioning of the liver, pancreas and spleen.
- ➤ Helps in dissolving gall bladder and kidney stones.
- ➤ Stimulates and promotes elimination of waste.
- ➤ Helps shrinking tumors.
- ➤ Treats effectively diarrhea and dysentery as it destroys harmful bacteria in the gut.
- ➤ Enhances night vision and promotes eye health.
- ➤ Treats effectively digestive problems such as heartburn, acidity and acid reflux.
- ➤ Heals burns, keeps the skin moisturized and youthful looking. Slows down the appearance of ageing signs.
- ➤ Improves lactation in nursing mothers.
- ➤ Treats earaches and improves hearing.
- ➤ Promotes heart health and prevents atherosclerosis.

Nutrition Information

Serving Size: 1 medium carrot (128g or 1 cup chopped carrot)

Percent Daily Values are based on a 2,000-calorie diet[1].

Calories		52	220kJ

Carbohydrates			
-	Total Carbohydrate	12.3g	4%
-	Dietary Fibre	3.6g	14%
-	Starch	1.8g	
-	Sugars	6.1g	

Fats and Fatty Acids		
-	Total Fat	0.3g
-	Saturated Fat	0.0g
-	Monounsaturated Fat	0.0g
-	Polyunsaturated Fat	0.1g
-	Total trans fatty acids	0.0g
-	Total Omega-3 fatty acids	2.6mg
-	Total Omega-6 fatty acids	147mg

Protein	1g

---

[1] http://nutritiondata.self.com/facts/vegetables-and-vegetable-products/2383/2

Vitamins

-	Vitamin A	21383IU42	8%
-	Vitamin C	7.6mg	13%
-	Vitamin E (Alpha Tocopherol)	0.8mg	4%
-	Vitamin K	16.9mcg	21%
-	Thiamin	0.1mg	6%
-	Riboflavin	0.1mg	4%
-	Niacin	1.3mg	6%
-	Vitamin B	60.2mg	9%
-	Folate	24.3mcg	6%
-	Vitamin B	120.0mcg	0%
-	Pantothenic Acid	0.3mg	3%
-	Choline	11.3mg	
-	Betaine	0.5mg	

Minerals

-	Calcium	42.2mg	4%
-	Iron	0.4mg	2%
-	Magnesium	15.4mg	4%
-	Phosphorus	44.8mg	4%
-	Potassium	410mg	12%
-	Sodium	88.3mg	4%
-	Zinc	0.3mg	2%
-	Copper	0.1mg	3%
-	Manganese	0.2mg	9%
-	Selenium	0.1mcg	0%
-	Fluoride	4.1mcg	

Sterols

-   Cholesterol 0mg   0.0mg   0%
-   Phytosterols   0.0mg   0%

Health Benefits

Carrots are among the most useful vegetables known to man, offering a goldmine of nutrients that promote the overall health of body and mind.

A few of the most important benefits are described below:

Improves Eyesight

The first thing anyone would tell you about the carrot is, *"it is good for the eyes."* The richest source of beta-carotene, carrots are indeed hugely beneficial for the health of the eyes. This compound promotes the production of Vitamin A, which in turn, transforms into a purple pigment named rhodopsin—a key compound for night vision in humans.

Beta-carotene is also a potent agent against macular degeneration and cataracts caused by ageing.

Lowers The Risk Of Cancer

Eating carrots on a regular basis will lower the risk of developing cancer by as much as one-third. It is especially beneficial against colon, breast and lung cancer. Falcarinol—a natural compound produced by the carrot—acts as a natural pesticide against fungal infection. The anti-cancer properties are derived from this compound.

Slows Ageing

One of the richest sources of antioxidants and Vitamin A, carrots fight against free radicals damage in the body and promotes repair and regeneration at cellular levels. The result is younger skin that looks radiant and fresh.

Besides preventing premature ageing and wrinkle formation, it helps in inhibiting and treating pigmentation, dry skin, acne and uneven skin tones.

Prevents Cardio Vascular Disease

Carrots are almost synonymous with beta-carotene—the compound that improves eyesight. However, carrots are also a rich source of antioxidants and other compounds such as alpha-carotene and lutein that prevent atherosclerosis and stroke by reducing the formation of cholesterol in the body and plaque in the arteries.

The soluble fibres in carrots have the ability to bind to the bile acids, thus reducing cholesterol to a large extent.

Respiratory Diseases

Carrots have the ability to clear mucus from lungs, ear, nose and throat areas. Hence, it can treat asthma, congestion and sinusitis. It also clears and prevents the damage that smoking and second-hand smoking cause the lungs.

Natural Cleanser

Carrots are one of the richest sources of Vitamin A, which is the key compound to help the liver expel toxins from the body. It also helps in reducing fat and bile in the liver. Packed with fibre, carrots also help treat constipation and promote the health of the colon by helping eliminate all waste.

Neonatal Jaundice

Drinking carrot juice during pregnancy would prevent neonatal jaundice in the newborn baby. It also boosts the immune system of the baby.

Rheumatism and Gout

The anti-inflammatory properties of carrots along with the ability to keep cholesterol in check are exceptionally beneficial for arthritic pain and gout.

Edema

Carrot juice is an excellent diuretic. It helps the body's excess water and is especially beneficial in reducing water retention in pregnant women and during menstruation.

Deworming

Just drinking one cup of carrot juice daily would get

rid of roundworms and pinworms.

Contraceptive

The seeds of the carrot prevent the ovum getting attached to the uterus. This is a well-known traditional method to prevent unwanted pregnancy.

Health Hazard

It is hard to imagine that this powerhouse of good nutrients has health downsides, as well. The common feeling about carrots is that when you introduce them into your life, you are signing a perfect health insurance policy.

Most of the downsides that you will find with the carrot happen only when this vegetable is eaten in excess. In moderation, there is only goodness and health coming from it. So, what are the health hazards that you may expect from the carrot?

Allergy

In very rare cases, people may find they are allergic to carrots. The symptoms of allergic reaction are a feeling of weakness, change in voice, and overall itchiness. The solution to people who have an allergy to carrots is to have them cooked.

Addiction

Carrots are known to be addictive in rare cases owing to a psychoactive compound named, "*myristicin*". However, to get addicted to carrots, you need to eat quite a lot of carrots every day.

Orange Colour Skin

When you eat too much of orange, red or yellow carrots, the beta-carotene content tends to show up in the skin. This is medically known as carotenoderma or caroteneia. It is most obvious in the face, palms, hands, and soles of the feet. The condition is totally harmless and it is reversed as soon as the carrot intake is reduced/ stopped.

Gas and Bloating

Consuming too many carrots would mean that you have a buildup of fibre, which can cause gas, bloating and stomach cramps.

CHAPTER 5: INTERESTING FACTS ABOUT CARROTS

Did You Know That ...?

... Both the words in the Latin name of the carrot, "Daucus Carota" mean orange?

... A rather little-known place in California by the name of Holtville has appropriated the title of "*Carrot Capital of the World*"? A festival is organized every year late January or early February?

... The carrot ranks second in popularity as a vegetable. The first place is taken by the potato?

... The flowers of carrots are known as Devil's Plague, Bees' Nest or Birds' Nest.

... In ancient days, carrots were cultivated exclusively for medicinal purposes?

... If you consume too much carrot, the skin turns orange owing to the carotene content of the carrot. The colour fades away once you reduce the intake of the vegetable. Babies are most susceptible to the skin colour change.

... Carrots come in all colours. Today you can have carrots that are black, purple, red, orange, yellow and white in colour. Take your pick?

... Orange carrots did not exist until the 16th century when they were developed in the Netherlands?

… Carrots are biennial vegetables. This means that you need two years to get seeds from this plant?

… The heaviest carrot in the world was produced in the USA; it weighed 8.44 kg (18.6 lb.)?

… The longest carrot in the world was produced in the United Kingdom; it measured 5.83 metres?

… Carrots contain the highest amount of carotene among all vegetables known to man. This compound converts to Vitamin A, which helps night sight in particular and eye health in general. Vitamin A also helps in preventing a number of cancers?

… Carrots are among the very few vegetables, which increase their nutrient powers on cooking. Most vegetables lose their nutrients on heating?

… That 1 glass of milk is equal to 9 carrots?

… The smallest of the baby carrots is called, "caroteenies"?

… You can run about 4.8 km on the power of just 3 carrots consumed?

… An adult American consumes about 12 pounds of carrots per year; about 3 pounds are in the form of canned or frozen, and 9 pounds are consumed fresh?

… There are about 100 varieties of carrots?

… Water makes for 88 percent of the carrot? The human body consists of 60 per cent water?

… As much as 85% of the total carrot produce in the

USA comes from Bakersfield, California?

... "Blushing" is the term used for the carrots on whose surface you see a white-ish coating. This indicates that the carrot is dehydrated owing to the peeling of the skin. To get the healthy-orange colour back, soak the carrot in ice-water for 2-3 minutes to get them hydrated.

... Carrots will have their flavour enhanced by certain spices such as thyme, tarragon, rosemary, raisins, orange, onion, honey, dill, curry, cumin, coriander, cinnamon, and chives.

... Carrot is a good companion plant. It co-exists well with chives, leeks and onions—which repel the greatest enemy of the carrot, the carrot root fly. The flower of the carrot attracts the predatory wasp, which is deadly to many gardening pests.

... Short carrots are sweeter? If you want your carrots less sweet, choose long ones.

... The maximum nutrients are just under the skin of the carrot? Hence, it is advised that you don't peel the carrot; rather rinse it thoroughly before you cook it or eat raw.

... Carrots were the first vegetables in the world to be canned?

... That the other names of the wild carrot are American carrot, rattlesnake weed, and Queen Anne's lace?

... Carrots decoction make excellent insecticide?

... If you place the carrot flowers in coloured water, the bloom will develop the colour of the water?

... The starling puts wild carrots in its nest? This helps kill the mites.

... The carrot leaves are eaten in Java?

...carrot oil is used in the perfumery industry and food flavouring and colouring?

... There is a superstition that if a girl brings in the flower of the carrot into the house, her mother will die?

Fun Facts About Carrots

➤ The carrot that Bugs Bunny chews on is a Denver variety.

➤ Mel Blanc, who lent his voice to Bugs Bunny, hated carrots.

➤ It is believed that if you dream of carrots, it means health and prosperity. If a young woman dreams she is eating carrots, it means she'll get married very soon.

➤ In Washington DC, it's illegal to distribute, sell, buy or transport carrot seeds. You may be fined up to $5,000 if caught doing any of these.

➤ In Europe it is believed that a gift of carrots to a newly-married couple brings luck to the bride in the kitchen.

➤ In many parts of the world, it is still believed that the carrot brings down sexual inhibitions in women.

CONCLUSION

Carrots are one of the most versatile vegetables today. Reading this eBook must have convinced you about this one fact. If you decide to add just one vegetable to your daily meals, it should be the carrot. This is not only a very tasty vegetable, which will complement any type of vegetable or meat, but also add a wealth of nutrients to each meal.

Try experimenting with this vegetable—not only the common and popular orange carrot, but also the black carrot, white carrot, yellow carrot and purple carrot. Have fun with the colours and tastes. Use it raw, blended in green smoothies, boiled, braised, broiled, baked, pickled, grilled and any other form you think of. This is a vegetable that tastes amazing in any form.

Here is wishing you a healthy, happy and long life!

Cheers!

USEFUL RESOURCES

Free eBooks And Useful Sites

1. How to grow carrots - https://www.rhs.org.uk/advice/grow-your-own/vegetables/carrots

2. Learn to grow carrots - http://www.extension.umn.edu/garden/yard-garden/vegetables/growing-carrots-and-root-vegetables/

3. Learn to grow carrots - http://www.motherearthnews.com/organic-gardening/learn-how-to-grow-carrots-zmaz08aszgoe.aspx

4. 146 Varieties of Carrots for Gardeners - http://vegvariety.cce.cornell.edu/main/showVarieties.php?searchCriteria=carrot&searchIn=1&crop_id=0&sortBy=overallrating&order=DESC

Free Videos

1. All About Carrots - http://www.foodnetwork.com/videos/all-about-carrots-0214964.html

Articles

1. Sweet and Bitter Taste in Organic Carrots - http://www.carrotmuseum.co.uk/Sweet%20and%20Bitter%20Taste%20in%20Organic%20Carrots.pdf

2. How to Cook Carrots - http://www.veg-world.com/articles/how-to-cook-carrots.htm

3. Vegan Coach - How to cook carrots - http://www.vegancoach.com/how-to-cook-carrots.html

Recipes

1. Carrot Jam - http://www.carrotmuseum.co.uk/jam.html

2. Carrot Marmalade - http://www.carrotmuseum.co.uk/marmalade.html

3. Carrot N Seaweed - http://realfoodforlife.com/carrots-with-arame/

4. Carrots N Orange - http://realfoodforlife.com/carrots-with-orange/

5. Carrot Chili - http://realfoodforlife.com/veganchili/

6. All types of recipes, which use carrot as a major

ingredient - http://allrecipes.com/recipes/fruits-and-vegetables/vegetables/carrots/

7. Recipes that use carrot - http://www.bbc.co.uk/food/carrot

8. Recipes with carrot - http://www.jamieoliver.com/recipes/vegetables-recipes/carrots/#ZCT2WwwJLIj3KFAb.97

9. Carrot cake recipes - http://www.gimmesomeoven.com/best-carrot-cake/

10. Carrot halwa recipe - http://www.vegrecipesofindia.com/gajar-halwa-recipe-carrot-halwa/

11. Carrot fudge (Indian sweet) - http://myheartbeets.com/carrot-fudge-indian-gajar-halwa-mithai/

12. 10 Best shredded carrot recipes - http://www.yummly.com/recipes/shredded-carrot-dessert

13. Carrot pudding recipe - http://www.thedomesticfront.com/carrot-pudding/

www.ingramcontent.com/pod-product-compliance
Lightning Source LLC
Chambersburg PA
CBHW050816290526
45792CB00001B/134